Wi
at**Weignt**LOSS

MW01046161

Proven strategies based on
diet, exercise & supplements

Sherry Torkos B.Sc. Phm.

ABOUT THE AUTHOR

As one of Canada's leading pharmacists, Sherry Torkos is well known for her knowledge and expertise in both conventional and complementary medicine. Sherry graduated with honors from the Philadelphia College of Pharmacy and Science in 1992. Since that time, she has been practicing pharmacy. She has won several national pharmacy awards for distinguished practice and for providing excellence in patient care.

Placing a strong emphasis on the role of nutrition, exercise and supplements in optimizing health and preventing disease, Sherry is active in providing educational programs for the public and other health care professionals. She is a certified fitness instructor and health enthusiast who enjoys sharing her passion with others.

Sherry is recognized in the media as an authority on health matters and is frequently featured on television and radio programs throughout North America.

She has authored several health booklets and numerous articles for both professional and consumer journals. In January 2003, she co-authored a book with Farid Wassef entitled, *Breaking the Age Barrier: Strategies for Optimum Health, Energy and Longevity*, published by Penguin Books.

For more information, visit her website: www.sherrytorkos.com

This booklet is intended for educational and informational purposes only. Please see a qualified medical professional if you have questions about your health.

First published in 2002 by Bearing Marketing Communications Inc.

If you have questions/comments about this book or are interested in bulk sales, etc., please contact Christiane Coté at John Wiley & Sons Canada, Ltd., 416-646-7992.

Production Credit

Cover Photograph by: Michael Dismatsek, Dismatsek Photographic, Burlington, ON
Cover Design and Interior Text Design by: Adrian So R.G.D.
Copy Editior/Proofreader: Nancy Carroll, Wordreach
Printer: Tri-Graphic Printing Ltd.

All product names and trademarks listed in this book are the property of their respective owners, including: Tonalin® CLA is a registered trade- mark of Natural Inc.; Endermologie® is a registered trademark of LPG Systems; Phase 2® is a trademark of Pharmachem Laboratories Inc.; Balance® is a registered trademark of Balance Bar Company; Genisoy® is a registered trademark of Genisoy Products Company; Luna Bar™ is a trademark of Clif Bar Inc.; Slim Down™ is a trademark of Jamieson Laboratories Inc.; Advantra Z® is a registered trademark of Nutratech, Inc.; NeOpuntia® is a registered trademark of Bio Serae Laboratories SA; COOL WHIP™ is a trademark of Kraft Foods Inc.

Printed in Canada
10 9 8 7 6 5 4 3 2

Table of Contents

TABLE OF CONTENTS

Foreword

FOREWORD

Over the last two decades North Americans have become a progressively fatter society. Each new fad diet highlights our rates of obesity, diabetes and heart disease, which have increased dramatically. According to the latest statistics, over a third of our children aged two to eleven are overweight and, of those, half could be considered obese. Knowing that diabetes, heart disease and certain cancers are directly linked to the amount of body fat we carry and the types of foods we eat, the prevalence of these diseases are expected to sky rocket.

The multi-billion-dollar diet industry with its no-fat, low-fat diets, sugar and fat substitutes, and prescription diet drugs and diet aids have done little to stop our waistlines from expanding.

Sherry Torkos has taken the science of fat loss and made it easy to apply to our everyday lives in this inspiring book. She provides cutting-edge information on the nutritional supplements that have been validated by clinical research to burn fat and increase metabolism.

Nutritional supplements are the cornerstone of Sherry's permanent weight-loss program. Scientifically proven nutrients are discussed at length for their fabulous weight-loss benefits. They include:

- Cassia Nomame, a fat blocker
- Citrus aurantium, a natural thermogenic

- conjugated linoleic acid, a fat that helps us burn fat
- green tea, a powerful thermogenic
- Phase 2®, a powerful starch blocker that allows us to eat the occasional dish of pasta and mashed potatoes.

For all those who are desperately dieting, the statistics show diets don't work. One year after dieting, 66 percent of people regain their weight, and after five years the figure rises to 97 percent. Simple lifestyle and diet changes provide the best results, and Sherry teaches you how to slim down, stay lean and live longer by adopting lifelong weight management strategies. Thyroid function, stress, hormones, genetics, serotonin, insulin, physical activity, the quality of our food not just how many calories we consume all have an effect on whether we lose weight or remain overweight.

Sherry's seven-day healthy meal plan will ensure you develop new eating habits and never feel hungry. *Winning at Weight Loss* is not just another diet book. It offers far more information and goes one step further by looking at health issues such as increased bone density, pain relief, sleep disturbances and mood enhancement. Even the causes and ways to eliminate cellulite are discussed.

Obesity will have the biggest financial impact on our health care systems in the future, if we don't move today to halt our increasing girth. I believe that this book can help you achieve your desired weight and optimal health in a safe manner.

Lorna R. Vanderhaeghe, B.Sc.
Author of the best-selling books *Healthy Immunity* and *The Immune System Cure,* and with co-author Karlene Karst, *Healthy Fats for Life*
www.healthyimmunity.com

Introduction
INTRODUCTION: The Obesity Epidemic

If you're struggling with your weight, you have plenty of company. Currently in the United States, over 60 percent of adults are overweight, and one-quarter are classified as obese. These figures represent an increase by over 50 percent in the last ten years alone. Approximately 48 percent of Canadian adults carry excess poundage and 15 percent are obese, according to the 2000/2001 Canadian Community Health Survey. There is no doubt that North America is in the midst of a serious obesity epidemic.

Being overweight is a risk factor for many chronic diseases, such as diabetes, heart disease and certain cancers. It also has far-reaching effects on a person's self-esteem and confidence. The good news is that, with the right tools, safe and long-term weight loss is possible—and it doesn't have to be painful. Forget what you have heard about the fad diets and gimmicks—they just don't work in the long run. In this booklet, you will learn how to adopt a fat-burning diet and rev up your metabolism through exercise. You will also find a no-nonsense view on the role of weight loss supplements—what works and what does not.

Desperate dieting

This prevalence of obesity is a paradox in our thinness-obsessed Western culture. Despite their collective girth, North Americans yearn to slim down and are willing to pay for it. A recent report from the Institute of Medicine (IOM) found that Americans spend more than $33 billion annually on weight reduction products, such as diet foods and drinks. The problem is that most of these "lose weight quick" products and schemes do not work. Very few have been clinically tested and some can even be hazardous to your health.

It is also ironic that despite this hefty expenditure, the rate of obesity has increased by more than 60 percent over the last ten years, and the future doesn't look any slimmer. Unfortunately, when dieters do lose weight, they usually gain it back, according to a panel of obesity, metabolic and other experts, who were convened by the National Institutes of Health (NIH). Studies show that one year after dieting, 66 percent of people regain their weight; after five years, that figure rises to 97 percent. Health authorities agree that in order to maintain long-term weight loss, you need to make long-term changes to your lifestyle. With these changes you will reap great health benefits—greater energy and vitality, and a reduced risk of chronic disease.

Obesity's impact on health

It is hard to escape the warnings from our national health agencies. The message they deliver is clear—obesity increases your risk of developing chronic disease. Jeffrey P. Coplan, director of the Centers for Disease Control and Prevention (CDC) states, "Obesity and overweight are linked to the nation's number-one killer—heart disease—as well as diabetes and other chronic conditions."

At a recent conference on obesity, held in Geneva, Switzerland, the World Health Organization (WHO) concluded, "Obesity's impact is so diverse and extreme that it should now be regarded as one of the greatest neglected public health problems of our time, with an impact on health which may well prove to be as great as that of smoking."

Just like smoking, obesity is one of the most preventable causes of chronic disease because in most cases its development is lifestyle-related. Taking in too many calories, eating unhealthy foods and not getting enough exercise are lifestyle choices— choices that can lead to serious consequences. Carrying extra weight is associated with increased blood pressure because the heart has to work harder. Having elevated blood pressure, known as hypertension, increases the risk of coronary heart disease and stroke. As well, diets that are high in fat and cholesterol contribute to an increased risk of coronary heart disease, gallstones and stroke.

Studies also show that overweight people are more susceptible to breast and colon cancers. Other health risks associated with obesity include post-surgical complications, delayed wound healing and an increased risk of infection and gout. Excess weight can put pressure on your lungs and chest, making it difficult to breathe and causing sleep apnea. It can also be stressful to the joints, back and hips leading to osteoarthritis, limited mobility, pain and discomfort. Overweight and obese women are at greater risk of having infertility and complications during childbirth.

The link between obesity and diabetes

One of the most talked about consequences of obesity today is the development of diabetes. In fact researchers have coined a new term for this association: *diabesity*. According to a report from the Centers for Disease Control, diabetes has officially reached epidemic proportions. Over 17 million Americans have diabetes, which represents a 49 percent increase in the past decade!

The two main forms of diabetes are Type 1 and Type 2. Type 1 is also known as insulin-dependent diabetes because the body loses the ability to produce insulin, leaving the individual reliant on regular injections of insulin to regulate blood sugar levels. This form of diabetes typically develops early in life, but it may also occur secondary to uncontrolled or advanced Type 2 diabetes.

Type 2 diabetes, which is also known as non-insulin dependent diabetes, is strongly associated with being overweight or obese, inactive and consuming a poor diet. This form of diabetes was previously associated with aging, but we are seeing it occur in many youth and children today because of their greater propensity toward obesity, lack of activity and poor eating habits.

The link between obesity and diabetes is quite strong—over 60 percent of people with Type 2 diabetes are obese. The reason for this is that obesity leads to the development of a condition called insulin resistance. Insulin is the hormone that is released from the pancreas in response to elevated blood sugar. When we eat, our food is broken down and digested, and the sugar that is absorbed from our meal causes our blood sugar level to rise. Insulin works to bring sugar (glucose) into the cell where it is used for energy, thus lowering our blood sugar. With insulin resistance, the body fails to respond properly to the insulin it already produces. As a result, blood sugar levels stay elevated and the body produces even more insulin in attempt to bring the sugar levels down. Yet, because the body is resistant to insulin, it is not able to lower blood sugar; therefore, it remains high. It is this inability to regulate blood sugar and insulin levels that is characteristic of Type 2 diabetes.

Researchers agree, the more weight you carry, the greater your chances of suffering from some or all of the conditions discussed above. This information should be taken as an incentive—to make the move today to work on developing a leaner, healthier body.

Childhood obesity

Sadly, young people represent the largest growing segment of the obese population. According to an estimate by the International Obesity Task Force, 22 million of the world's children under five years of age are overweight or obese. In the United States, obesity rates in children have almost tripled in the past 25 years. The most recent government numbers available show the percentage of kids ages six to 18 who were overweight increased to 15 percent in 1999–2000 from 6 percent in the late 1970s.

The picture is worse in Canada. A long-term study of Canadian children revealed one of the highest rates of childhood obesity in the world. At least one in four is overweight, compared to one in ten when the study began in 1981. Unfortunately, this trend is also being seen in other areas of the world such as Europe, Australia and the Caribbean.

The obesity epidemic is having far-reaching effects on the health of our children. A recent study found one in eight children have three or more risk factors for what doctors call metabolic syndrome, a cluster of symptoms that serve as an early warning signal for heart disease and diabetes. And more than half of the children have at least one of the risk factors. These risk factors include high blood pressure, inefficient processing of glucose, elevated insulin levels, low levels of "good" HDL cholesterol and elevated triglycerides—a fatty substance found in the blood.

Overweight children are at risk of becoming obese adults, and obese adults are at greater risk for raising obese children, and so the cycle continues.

Costs to society

Obesity is not only hard on health—it is hard on the national pocketbook. The health-related costs of treating obesity are estimated at $117 billion per year in the United States alone.

The psychosocial effects of being overweight may be as serious as the hazards to physical health. As unfounded as this may be, North American society has a strong bias against overweight people, typically stigmatizing them as bad, lazy, ugly and lacking will power. Surveys of children as young as kindergarten age indicate that negative perceptions about obesity begin very early in life. Children believe that their obese peers are not as clean or as smart as other children. Unfortunately, these attitudes pervade our society, creating discrimination against the obese.

Lose weight and live longer

According to a recent report from the U.S. Surgeon General, obese individuals have a 50 to 100 percent greater risk of premature death from all causes than individuals without excess weight. An estimated 300,000 deaths are attributed to obesity in the United States each year.

Controlling your weight may extend your life span, according to research published in the *Journal of the American Medical Association* (JAMA). This study looked at body weight and mortality in a group of 19,000 middle-aged men over the course of 27 years. Researchers found that the men who were lean lived significantly longer than those who were extremely under- or overweight. This is no surprise, considering the effects that excess weight has on your risk of developing chronic disease.

It may be comforting to know that even small losses can result in great health rewards. If you are overweight, losing even 5 to 10 percent of that excess can dramatically improve your health—lowering y ol level and blood sugar. Plus, y el motivated to continue with yo

DEFINING OB

There are a variety of her you are carrying excess weight h problems. The easiest and most common method is the body mass index (BMI). The BMI is a mathematical formula that is highly correlated with body fat and which has gained international acceptance.

The BMI represents your weight in pounds, divided by your height in inches squared. Here is how you calculate it in imperial measurements:

1. Multiply your weight, in pounds, by 0.45. For example, if you weigh 140 lbs.: 140 x 0.45 = 63

2. Multiply your height, in inches, by 0.025. For example, if you are 5 ft. 6 in. (66 inches): 66 x 0.025 = 1.65
3. Square the answer from step 2: 1.65 x 1.65 = 2.72
4. Divide the answer from step 1 by the answer from step 3: 63 / 2.72 = 23.16

Refer to Table 2 on page 59 to determine your BMI.

If your BMI is under 18.5, you may be underweight. If your BMI falls between 18.5 and 24.9—as is the case in the example above—your weight is likely within normal range. If your BMI is over 25, you are probably overweight. If it is over 30, you are likely obese.

A drawback of the BMI is that it neither distinguishes fat from muscle, nor takes into account the higher body fat content normally found in females. Using this method, a body builder could appear to be obese because of a greater muscle mass (muscle weighs more than fat).

Another method of checking your health risk is the waist-to-hip ratio, which reflects the proportion of body fat located around the abdomen. An apple-shaped body (large abdomen) is more often linked to health problems, such as heart disease and cancer. Having a waist-to-hip ratio greater than 0.95 for men and 0.80 for women is associated with increased health risks.

Because body composition (fat versus muscle) is a more important factor in determining health risks, the preferred method is to check your percentage of body fat. This can be done with fat calipers or a bioelectric impedance device. Using this method, men with more than 25 percent and women with more than 30 percent body fat are considered to be obese.

Target Body Fat Ranges:
Women 15–25%
Men 10–20%

CAUSES OF OBESITY AND WEIGHT GAIN

In the past, the first law of thermodynamics was often used to explain the control of body weight. Simply put, if energy intake (food) exceeds energy expenditures (exercise/activity), then weight gain occurs. Conversely, reducing intake and increasing expenditures was believed to be the key to weight loss. For years, doctors and researchers believed this simple theory to be the answer. We now know, however, that other factors are involved. Some people can exercise religiously, reduce food intake and still not lose weight. And, of course, we all know people who can eat whatever they want and never gain a pound.

Weight gain and obesity are complex conditions, dependent upon various lifestyle, hormonal, biochemical, metabolic and genetic factors. Some of the most important factors include:

Basal Metabolic Rate (BMR) Your BMR rate at which your body burns calories at rest. This rate is dependent on several of the factors listed below, such as activity level and thyroid function.

Caloric intake Overeating and consuming more calories than your body uses for energy can result in weight gain—regardless of whether those calories come from fat, carbohydrates or protein.

Quality of food Eating too much saturated fat, sugar, processed food and fast food is associated with weight gain.

Physical activity Your activity level is the major player in weight balance. Inactivity causes loss of muscle mass, a reduced metabolic rate and increased body fat. Conversely, regular exercise can improve muscle mass and boost metabolism. As we exercise, our muscles utilize calories for energy and generate heat, which promotes the burning of fat.

Stress Exposure to chronic stress can cause weight gain, particularly around the mid-section. This occurs because stress increases the production and release of cortisol, a hormone that increases body fat storage.

Thyroid function The thyroid gland plays a vital role in controlling metabolism. If your thyroid is sluggish and not functioning optimally, this can reduce your metabolic rate and cause weight gain.

Insulin When insulin levels are high, the body stores more fat and is not able to use fat as a source of energy—the reason insulin is also known as "the fat storage hormone." This can be a problem for those with insulin resistance who often develop hyperinsulinemia (high insulin levels).

Genetics Genetics may be responsible for about 25 percent of obesity cases, but experts agree that having a genetic predisposition towards obesity does not mean that this is your fate. Several studies have shown that lifestyle factors are a more important determinant.

Estrogen High estrogen levels are associated with weight gain. Yet, many women find that they gain weight during menopause while their estrogen levels are lower. This happens because as estrogen levels decline in menopause, as a compensatory mechanism, the fat cells take over the production of estrogen. In order to meet the growing demand during menopause, they increase in size and number.

Testosterone Testosterone helps the body maintain lean muscle mass and burn fat. A deficiency of this hormone can cause the loss of muscle mass and fat gain. This is a significant contributor to fat gain in older men.

Human growth hormone (HGH) By increasing lean muscle mass and reducing body fat storage, human growth hormone regulates body weight. Levels decline with age, particularly after age 50, causing a shift in our body composition. As HGH decreases, we gain body fat and lose muscle mass.

Serotonin Serotonin is a chemical messenger in the brain that regulates satiety. When levels are low, we feel hungry and when they are high, we feel satisfied. Certain weight-loss products work by elevating serotonin to promote satiety and reduce cravings for food.

Leptin Satiety is also regulated by leptin, a hormone produced by body fat. Researchers have found that some people become resistant to their own leptin. To compensate for this the body produces more and more of the hormone, but the "satisfied" message is not property received by the brain.

The carbohydrate conundrum

The latest movement in the diet industry is the avoidance of carbs. The over-consumption of carbohydrate foods leading to problems with blood sugar balance and obesity has become the focus of many new weight loss books, diets and supplements.

Before carbohydrates became the enemy, the focus was on fats. The anti-fat movement began in the 1980s. Studies and health reports warned us of the dangers of consuming diets high in fat—obesity, heart disease and cancer. In response to this many individuals cut down on consuming foods high in fat or avoided them completely. Surprisingly, this movement did not result in weight loss. In fact we became even fatter. The reason for this is that we did not cut down our caloric intake; we shifted our calories from fats to carbohydrates, particularly the starchy and sugary forms, and also increased our portion sizes. Reports issued by the United States Department of Agriculture (USDA) show that total caloric intake has steadily increased over the past few decades. In 1970, we consumed an average of 3,300 calories per day. In 1995, that number jumped to more than 3,800 calories. These same reports show that carbohydrate consumption has increased over the past 30 years, along with obesity rates.

To understand the link between carbohydrates and weight gain, it is important to understand how these foods are digested. When carbohydrates are consumed, enzymes in the digestive tract break these large molecules into smaller sugar molecules. These sugars are absorbed through the intestine and then either burned for energy or stored as fat. If the body consumes more of these calories than it burns during exercise and activity, the excess gets stored as fat.

One reason carbohydrate consumption has increased is that these foods are convenient, easy to prepare and satisfying to the palate. We have toast, bagels or muffins for breakfast, bread or pasta for lunch, and rice or potatoes for dinner. And some of us are eating two to four starch servings per meal or more. Would you believe that one jumbo New York-style bagel represents five servings of carbohydrate! Portion sizes have certainly changed over the past few decades. Prior to the carbohydrate boom of the 1980s, muffins and bagels were about two ounces. Today, muffins are six to eight ounces and bagels are as high as ten ounces.

Carbohydrates are an important part of a healthful diet—they provide a readily available source of energy and are rich in vitamins, minerals and fiber. The problem is that our intake of carbohydrates has sky-rocketed and we are eating too many of the wrong types of carbohydrates—those high in refined sugars and flours. These foods, which include bagels, muffins, cookies, pasta, white bread, potatoes and rice, pack a lot of calories and are high on the glycemic index (GI).

The GI is a scale that measures the impact of different foods on our blood sugar levels. The scale spans from 0 to 100, with 100 being the GI of pure glucose. Foods that are rapidly broken down and absorbed into our blood stream, such as sugar, refined grains (white bread and rice) and potatoes, cause a rapid increase in blood sugar and therefore have a higher GI, in the range of 70 to 100. In general, foods that are high in fiber, such as whole grains and vegetables, have a lower GI. Foods that are classified as having a low glycemic index have a rating of 50 or less. Eggs, meats, dairy products and other proteins also have a low GI. Refer to Table 1 on page 58 for the Glycemic Index of common foods.

Eating foods with a high glycemic index causes a rapid increase in blood glucose and insulin levels. This is taxing to the pancreas and can cause mood swings, foggy head and weakness. Since high insulin levels can cause the body to store more fat, foods with a high GI (even if they are carbohydrates) can contribute to weight gain and obesity.

LIFELONG WEIGHT MANAGEMENT STRATEGIES

Researchers continually seek a greater understanding of obesity, so they can develop more effective strategies for treating it. In the meantime, we must realize that there is no "magic bullet" for weight loss. Instead, we need to develop a comprehensive strategy that includes a balanced diet, consistent exercise and safe supplementation. Our day-to-day choices will make far more difference to our weight and overall health than any other single factor. We can't afford to ignore the health consequences of obesity. We need to take steps now to adopt a healthier lifestyle. Keep in mind that even small losses lead to great health rewards—reduced blood pressure, sugar and cholesterol levels along with overall improved well-being.

Dietary guidelines

A healthy, balanced diet is key for weight management. Many of us think we are doing okay, yet according to the USDA, 80 percent of Americans do not eat a healthy diet. Worse yet, only one percent of children are eating a healthy diet. Clearly, there is a lack of knowledge and understanding of what constitutes a healthy diet.

In 2000 the U.S. government released a report on new dietary guidelines. This was the first time in nearly 30 years that changes had been recommended. Among these recommendations was a greater emphasis on eating whole grains, fruits and vegetables. They also proposed changes to the recommendation for macronutrient (protein, carbohydrates and fat) balance. In order to meet the body's daily energy and nutritional needs while minimizing risk for chronic disease, it was recommended that adults should receive:

- 45 to 65 percent of their calories from carbohydrates
- 20 to 35 percent from fat
- 10 to 35 percent from protein.

Since carbohydrates, fat and protein all serve as energy sources and provide calories, these ranges should be used as a guideline for menu planning. "We established ranges for fat, carbohydrates and protein because they must be considered together," said panel chair Joanne Lupton, a professor of nutrition at Texas A&M University, College Station. "Studies show that when people eat very low levels of fat combined with very high levels of carbohydrates, high-density lipoprotein concentration, or 'good' cholesterol decreases," and this is undesirable. "Conversely, high-fat diets can lead to obesity and its complications if caloric intake is increased as well, which is often the case. We believe these ranges will help people make healthy and more realistic choices based on their own food preferences."

In terms of the recommended caloric intake, it varies depending on height, weight, gender and activity level. For example, a 30-year-old woman who is 5 feet 5 inches tall and weighs 111 to 150 pounds should consume between 1,800 and 2,000 calories daily if she lives a sedentary lifestyle. However, if she is a very active person, her recommended total caloric intake increases to 2,500 to 2,800 calories per day. If her lifestyle fits the moderately active category as defined in the report, which is the minimum level of activity to decrease risk of chronic disease, she should eat between 2,200 and 2,500 calories daily. Using grams for the recommended ranges of intake, she should consume 55 to 97 grams of fat and 285 to 375 grams of carbohydrates per day.

Experts agree that healthy eating rather than restrictive dieting is the best way to lose weight and keep it off. Here are my top nutritional tips to consider for achieving a healthy body weight:

1. Eat at least three meals a day, preferably four to five small meals to keep your metabolism and energy level optimized. Do not skip meals as this can raise your appetite, deplete your energy levels and lead to binge eating. When you are hungry between meals, snack on healthful foods, such as fruit, yogurt, raw vegetables, nuts and seeds.

2. Emphasize fresh, unprocessed foods. Low-fat, nutrient-dense foods are your best dietary choices. These include fresh fruits, vegetables, legumes (beans, peas and lentils) and whole grains. Cut down on processed and refined foods, such as fast food, junk food, white bread, rice and pasta, candy, cookies and sweets. Refined grains lack nutritional value because their outer fiber-rich layer is stripped away during the refinement. Processed food and junk food should be looked upon as providing "empty calories" because these foods are often high in sugar and calories but very low in nutritional value. If you enjoy these foods, reserve them as a special treat and work on minimizing your serving size.

3. Eat a variety of wholesome foods. This is the best way to ensure you get the optimum amount of vitamins, minerals and phyto-

chemicals you need to support lifelong health. We have a tendency to eat the same foods over and over. By doing this we miss out on some of the nutrients provided by eating different foods.

4. Incorporate more fat-fighting foods into your diet, such as soy and flaxseed. Soy foods can improve fat metabolism. The phytoestrogens in soy (plant-based estrogen-like substances) bind to estrogen receptors in the body, reducing the amount of fat that enters the fat cells. Flaxseed contains dietary fiber, and also provides a rich source of lignans. Lignans have been shown to inhibit aromatase—an enzyme in body fat which converts testosterone into estrogen. High estrogen levels are a factor in weight gain. By preventing this conversion, lignans help to balance hormone levels and may play a role in controlling hormone-related weight gain.

5. Limit your intake of saturated and hydrogenated fats. Fat fills you up more slowly than other foods because it takes longer to metabolize and absorb from the gastrointestinal tract. The feeling of fullness (satiety) is delayed, causing you to eat more. Less chewing is required, so these fatty foods are consumed quickly. Furthermore, fat is more calorie-dense, providing nine calories per gram compared to only four calories per gram provided by protein and carbohydrates.

   Be aware that many of the new fat-free products on the market use sugar to replace the fat, providing just as many calories as the original product. Consider the following:

   • A serving of Lite Cool Whip™ contains the same number of calories as the regular kind: 25 calories per two tablespoons.
   • A cup of non-fat vanilla yogurt has 223 calories, while the whole-milk version has only 24 calories more.
   • Putting two tablespoons of jelly on a bagel instead of a tablespoon of butter gets rid of the fat but does not reduce

the number of calories because of the sugar content. While we need to watch our intake of saturated and hydrogenated fats, it is important not to cut out the good fats (essential fatty acids), which are found in fish, nuts, seeds and vegetables. Essential fatty acids are *essential* for health. They are important for proper function of the brain, heart and each cell in our body.

6. Ensure adequate protein intake. Protein is essential for building and maintaining lean muscle mass. Without adequate protein intake, dieting and exercise can cause the body to burn muscle for fuel and this can result in a lowering of your basal metabolic rate—the rate at which you burn calories. The recommended amount of protein is based on body weight and activity level. For the average person, this amount is 0.8 to 1 gram per kilogram of body weight. For example, if you weigh 63 kilograms, your total protein intake should be about 50 to 63 grams. Focus on eating lean protein, such as poultry, fish, eggs, nuts and seeds. Red meat is okay in moderation as long as you trim the fat and watch your portion sizes. If you can't get enough protein in your diet, consider a supplement.

   There are many products on the market which vary greatly in taste, formulation and quality. My recommendation is to choose a product that provides at least 20 grams per serving and is low in carbohydrate and free of artificial ingredients and sweeteners. Protein powders can be used to make shakes in the morning or between meals. My top recommended brands are listed in Table 4 on page 60.

7. Fill up on fiber. Dietary fiber is a powerful asset to anyone trying to lose body fat. Dietary fiber helps balance blood sugar and insulin levels and improves digestion and elimination. Fiber also makes us feel more full with meals because it slows digestion.

Unfortunately, most North Americans only consume about 10 to 15 grams of fiber daily. Health authorities, including The National Cancer Institute and the Institute of Medicine recommend 25 to 35 grams of fiber per day. Plant foods, such as vegetables, fruit, whole grains and legumes are excellent sources of natural fiber. Fiber is also available in supplemental form, such as powders and tablets. Read your labels carefully to ensure that you are getting a good quality product that delivers a reasonable amount of fiber per serving. When increasing your fiber intake, do so gradually. You may notice some temporary gas or bloating as you boost your fiber intake. This is common and should not deter you. Make sure that you drink plenty of water (8 to 10 glasses) each day. For a list of recommended fiber supplements, refer to page 60.

8. If you drink alcoholic beverages, do so in moderation. Alcohol floods the body with empty calories. Depending on the beverage, it provides anywhere from 20 to 124 calories per ounce.

9. Cut down on salt and sodium. Most of the sodium in the North American diet comes from the salt shaker and processed foods. A high-sodium diet is unhealthy and causes fluid retention, meaning it can contribute to water weight gain.

10. Consider taking a well-balanced multivitamin/mineral formula. As you are reducing your calorie intake, you may also be reducing your nutrient intake. A high-quality multivitamin can help fill any dietary gaps.

Nutritional deficiencies are not only hard on your health—they are also hard on your weight-loss program because they can cause food cravings and binge eating. Nutritionist and author Patrick Quillin, Ph.D., R.D., C.N.S., explains that addressing nutritional imbalances is the key to controlling appetite. Dr. Quillin writes, "A number of binge eaters are deficient in some nutrients, and they devour everything in sight in their hunger for that nutrient." Folic acid, vitamins A, B6, B12 and C, thiamin, niacinamide and riboflavin are some of the nutrients that influence appetite.

When working properly, the appetite is like a Geiger counter, seeking a reasonable amount of total calories and a proper mix of protein, carbohydrate and fat. People who do not get enough fat and protein end up ravenously hungry. As a result, they fill up on junk food (salty, sugary, starchy foods) in search of these key macronutrients.

Importance of water

One of the most important dietary tips I can suggest is to drink at least eight eight-ounce glasses of pure water daily. Water plays many vital roles in health. While you are losing weight, toxins stored in the fat tissue are released into your bloodstream. Drinking plenty of pure water makes it easier for your liver and kidneys to cope with the breakdown of toxins. Water also works with fiber to keep your bowels regular and prevent constipation. Having a glass before and during meals can help fill you up and reduce the quantity of food consumed.

Anthony Conte, M.D., a physician who specializes in bariatrics (a branch of medicine that focuses on obesity and related conditions), states, "By drinking water and correcting fluid retention, more fat is used as fuel because the liver is free to metabolize fat at top speed."

Dr. Conte also makes the following points about water:

• If you do not drink enough water, the body feels threatened. In self-protection, it will hoard every molecule of water in the body, leading to fluid retention and bloating.

- Drinking plenty of water helps protect against the sagging skin that may otherwise occur during fat loss.
- Heavy people need more water than thin people because they have a larger metabolic burden. Drinking water is critical for weight loss and for supporting good health during the stress of lifestyle changes.

Beware of fad diets

Apparently, the North American public never tires of fad diets. Each week there seems to be a new diet program or plan promoted in the tabloids. Promises for quick results and celebrity endorsements give us hope and the belief that these plans will work for us. Unfortunately many of these diets are not backed by science, and some can be dangerous to your health. For example, a recent diet I came across promotes that you can lose ten pounds in two days by consuming a liquid tonic of various herbs and nutrients. No food is allowed, or any liquids other than water for the two days. No doubt, a two-day fast will result in some weight loss. Since the product contains herbs with diuretic properties, water loss will also occur. It is important to realize however, that this type of weight loss is temporary and can be dangerous, especially for those with diabetes, or kidney or heart problems. Once you start eating and drinking fluids again, the weight will come back.

Stay away from diets that are drastically low in calories (less than 800 calories per day). While these diets can lead to rapid weight loss, they can be dangerous to your health. Restrictive diets cause the body to cannibalize (break down) its own muscle for fuel, causing muscle-wasting, which reduces metabolism. These diets also induce nutrient deficiencies, and over the long term, may result in starvation, organ failure and death.

While many fad diets come and go, one that has been around for decades and continuing to grow in popularity is the low-carb, high-protein diet promoted by Dr. Robert Atkins and others. When this diet was first introduced in the 1970s it was met with great skepticism among the mainstream medical community. There were concerns about its safety and efficacy. Initially there was little research to back the claims. The rationale was based on theory and a few small studies.

Now a growing number of studies have shown that a low-carb, high-protein diet can not only facilitate greater weight loss, but can also deliver benefits for reduction of heart disease. Several of the studies evaluating the effects of these diets have found improvement in risk factors for heart disease. Specifically, it has been demonstrated that the low-carb, high-protein diets can raise good cholesterol (HDL), lower bad cholesterol (LDL) and reduce triglycerides. This type of diet is challenging to follow and is definitely not for everyone.

If you decide to follow a low-carb, high-protein diet, here are some points to keep in mind:

- Eating a diet of primarily protein and fat will keep you satisfied longer and help curb cravings, so you will consume fewer calories overall.
- When you first begin a low-carb, high-protein diet, the weight loss will be more dramatic because you will be losing primarily water weight.
- Excessive protein intake can leach calcium out of your bones and be stressful to the kidneys. Most of these diets, such as Atkins, recommend a higher but not excessive intake of protein; however, it is important to drink lots of water and to be monitored by your doctor.
- It is important to take a good quality multivitamin and mineral supplement along with essential fatty acids and fiber while following this type of diet to make up for what is not obtained through the diet due to restriction of carbohydrates.

Avoid the fat-free frenzy

Although the popularity of the fat free diets has faded, there are still some misconceptions about fat. Fats are not all bad. In fact, the good fats are important for health and can even influence body weight. The problem is that we are consuming too many of the bad fats—the saturated and trans-fatty acids and not nearly enough of the essential fatty acids (EFAs).

EFA deficiencies are common in North America, yet they are so critical for health. EFAs are incorporated into all the cells in our body. They are important components of hormone-like compounds that help control blood pressure, decrease cholesterol levels and reduce body fat. Good sources of EFAs include conjugated linoleic acid, flaxseed oil, nuts, fish oil, evening primrose oil, black currant oil and borage oil.

Extra virgin olive oil is also considered a "good" fat. In countries where people consume olive oil, even in high amounts, they have lower rates of chronic diseases such as heart disease, certain cancers, osteoporosis, cataracts, arthritis, gallbladder disease, hypertension and stroke.

Just as we need some fat in our diet, we also need some (but not too much) body fat for cushioning. Fatty tissue supplies reserve energy as well as padding around the nerve plexus and abdominal organs. The body needs stores of fat and other nutrients to draw upon during times of stress and starvation.

Fast food is bad food

It is no surprise that the fast food industry is booming, right along with the rising rates of obesity. Fast food outlets spend billions of dollars each year on consumer advertising—enticing you to purchase those meals laden with fat, sugar and empty calories. Over the past 40 years, fast food has drastically changed the experience of dining out in North America and around the world. You do not even have to get out of your car; you can drive up, pick up your order and drive away as you eat on the run.

Fast food is cheap, quick and convenient. With the availability of big portions of fries and colas, many consumers feel they are getting a deal. However, did you know that a super-sized order of fries provides 540 calories and 26 grams of fat? And a large 32-ounce cola packs 310 calories? Unfortunately, that "deal" translates into extra body fat and an increased risk of obesity-related conditions.

Eating fast food once a week or less is probably not going to do you irreparable harm. However, if fast food is a staple of your diet, and fresh, unprocessed foods are the exception, then it is time to reverse this unhealthy habit.

When you do go to a fast-food establishment, choose the healthier items: grilled chicken, veggie burger or salad with dressing on the side, instead of chicken nuggets, a fried fish sandwich, large and jumbo-size fries, sauces and high-fat add-ons such as cheese, chili and tartar sauce.

PHYSICAL ACTIVITY IS ESSENTIAL FOR WEIGHT LOSS

Lack of physical activity is a major factor in our obesity epidemic. Modern life offers fewer opportunities for burning calories. Children watch more television and spend more time playing computer games; many schools have reduced or eliminated physical education classes; many neighborhoods lack sidewalks for safe walking; the workplace has become increasingly automated; and walking and cycling have been replaced by automobile travel.

According to a recent survey only 34 percent of obese individuals participate in moderate physical activity. Clearly, a lack of exercise is fueling this epidemic.

Keep in mind, to control weight you need to exercise, and exercise can be fun! You can certainly reduce your weight by reducing your calorie intake. But by adding a 30-minute brisk walk four days a week, you can double your rate of weight loss. Boost that to five days a week and the rewards are greater. Those who work out five times a week have been found to lose three times as much fat as those who exercise only two or three times weekly.

The guidelines released from the National Academies Institute of Medicine recommend that, regardless of weight, adults and children should also spend a total of at least one hour each day in moderately intense physical activity. This is double the daily goal set by the 1996 Surgeon General's report, and takes into consideration the increased caloric intake of our population, our lack of activity and our rising prevalence of obesity.

Two of the most common reasons people give for not exercising are—*lack of time* and *can't afford*. We all seem to have very busy lifestyles and put exercise at the bottom of our list of priorities, while it should be near the top. There are so many ways that we can incorporate moderate physical activity into our daily lifestyle. Doing housework or gardening with vim and vigor, washing your car (instead of using the drive-through), dancing and brisk walking are just some examples of activities that we can work into our day with no cost. If you can't fit an hour in, then try to spend a half hour in the morning and half hour in the evening. Every little bit helps.

Consistent exercise promotes the loss of body fat in several ways:

- **Increased energy expenditures** Exercise or physical activity burns calories and stored fat. Even if you continue to eat exactly as you do now, and start exercising consistently, you can lose 30 pounds over the next year.
- **Afterburn** Your basal metabolic rate is heightened for four to 24 hours after vigorous physical activity.
- **Increased lean body mass** Exercise is critical for building and maintaining strong, healthy muscles and muscle burns more calories than any other part of the body. Increasing lean muscle mass helps the body to utilize fat

more efficiently as fuel. Dieting without exercise can actually undermine your weight-loss efforts by leading to loss of muscle mass along with fat. When this happens metabolism slows down and you burn fewer calories.

- **Slowing down the movement of food through your digestive tract** Physical activity helps control your weight by slowing down the digestive process. Since your stomach takes longer to empty, you feel full longer.
- **Balancing blood sugar** Exercise pulls stored calories, or energy, in the forms of glucose and fat out of tissues. In this way, blood glucose levels stay balanced and you are less likely to feel hungry.

As I discussed earlier, being active daily is not only recommended, but essential for overall health. If you are interested in taking your weight loss program a step further and want to maximize fat loss, then it is important to consider a regular exercise program that includes a combination of aerobic (cardiovascular) activity, toning/strength training and stretching.

Contrary to popular belief, doing aerobic activity alone is not the most effective way to lose body fat. Aerobic activities (walking, biking, dancing, etc.) do burn calories and provide health benefits, but resistance training (i.e., weight lifting) plays an even stronger role in weight loss because it boosts your metabolism, improves thermogenesis (calorie-burning) and promotes loss of body fat. These exercises build lean muscle mass. Remember, the more muscle you have, the more calories you burn. In fact, one pound of muscle burns roughly 50 calories per day, compared to one pound of fat, which burns only two to three calories per day.

Resistance training is particularly important for adults because it helps slow down the muscle loss that occurs with aging. For those of you who are in your 40s you may have noticed the undesirable shift in body composition that happens with age.

We start to lose our muscle mass and gradually gain body fat, especially around the mid-section. Another benefit of resistance training is that it improves balance, increases endurance and improves bone density (reducing the risk of osteoporosis).

To create an effective program, choose a balance of activities, in a particular order. It was previously thought that cardio exercises should be done first, to allow the muscles to warm up and to maximize fat loss. However, during the first 20 minutes of your workout, sugar (carbohydrate), rather than fat, is the primary source of fuel. So, in order to burn fat calories with aerobic activities, you have to do more than 20 minutes of that activity. Unfortunately, most people do not have the time to spend more than 20 minutes on the treadmill or bike. Many sports researchers feel that it is much better to do cardio after your weight-training routine. This way, our bodies will be switched into fat-burning mode and you can take advantage of the endorphins and hormones (testosterone and growth hormone) that are released after your weight workout.

For optimal cardiovascular (and fat-burning) benefits, your aerobic program should bring your heart rate up to 60 to 80 percent of your maximum rate for 30 minutes at least four times a week. To find out what that rate is, subtract your age from 220; then calculate 60 to 80 percent of that figure.

Here are some exercise recommendations to enhance fat loss and improve body composition.

Resistance training
Goal: Work out with weights for 20 to 40 minutes every other day

Exercises: Choose two body parts per workout. For example, chest and triceps on Monday, back and biceps on Wednesday, and legs and shoulders on Friday. Vary your exercises and routine to challenge the muscles. Pick two exercises per body part and do two to three sets of that move. For example, do chest presses and dumbbell flies to work the chest. Start off by using a lower weight and doing 15 to 20 repetitions of each move. Over a period of several weeks, increase the weight and lower the repetitions, so you are using a weight that fatigues your muscle in eight to 12 repetitions.

Tips: Take the time to do the move properly. Bad technique can lead to injury and make workouts less effective. Be consistent—do not miss a workout. Find a partner for motivation and consistency. Seek the advice of a personal trainer to learn how to use the weights and machines properly.

Cardiovascular activity
Goal: 30 to 45 minutes, five times per week

Exercises: Examples of cardiovascular activities include walking, swimming, biking, aerobics, dancing and inline skating. Start slowly and gradually increase the duration and intensity of your activities. If you can only do five minutes to start, that is fine. With time, endurance improves.

Tips: Pick activities that you enjoy and try to do them first thing in the morning or right after work, preferably on an empty stomach. To increase intensity, add power to the movements. For example, when a brisk 30-minute walk can be done with ease, add hand/ankle weights or travel on an incline.

It is best to exercise on an empty stomach, or after a light snack or protein shake. Try to fit in your workouts in the morning, since you have more energy and will continue to burn calories for several hours afterward. If you can't exercise in the morning, then try to go during your lunch hour.

Before a weight routine, warm up with a walk or bike for five to ten minutes, and do a set of light weights first to increase blood flow to the muscles and get yourself warmed up. After the workout, remember to stretch. This will help prevent soreness the next day, and is a great way to relax and cool down.

In the past, stretching was recommended before a workout to reduce your risk of injury and muscle strain. The latest research, however, found that this is not the case. Australian researchers reviewed five studies on the effects of stretching and muscle soreness, and found that it offered no benefits before a workout. However, stretching is not a waste of time—it does help improve flexibility, increase blood flow and relieve pain after a workout. Stretching can also be a relaxing way to end your day and helps to work out tension and knots in the muscles. Take your time when doing a stretch and hold the position for at least ten seconds to get the most benefits.

Beginners, start slowly

If you have been sedentary all your life, the prospect of getting active may be intimidating. The most important advice for beginners is to take it slowly. Getting into shape is a gradual, incremental process. If you do too much too soon, you may injure yourself or become too discouraged to continue.

Start by taking a five-minute walk around the block, to your friend's house or a store. The next day, walk six or seven minutes. Day by day, steadily increase the time and intensity of your activity. You will build your capacity for physical activity, making it easier to push yourself to the next level.

Make sure you find activities you enjoy, because you are not as likely to stick with something that is not fun. You may need to try a number of activities to find one or two you like. It may be walking, lifting weights, swimming or water exercises, bicycling, racquetball, tennis, dancing, rowing, yoga, kick-boxing or aerobics classes. It may be a combination of any of the above. Remember, activities such as raking leaves, playing with young children, gardening and housework also contribute to greater fitness and weight control.

Other benefits of exercise

In addition to weight control, consistent physical activity offers the following impressive benefits:

1. **Improved mood** Even light exercise can boost your emotional well-being. Aerobic exercise stimulates the release of certain mood-elevating compounds called endorphins— "feel good" chemicals. These natural painkillers induce relaxation and relieve depression.

2. **Reduced risk of heart disease** If you are overweight, you face a higher risk of cardiovascular disease. In a study conducted at Washington University School of Medicine in St. Louis, a group of individuals participated in an exercise program. After 12 months of endurance workouts, their cardiovascular function improved by 25 to 30 percent. Exercise can also effectively lower blood pressure and cholesterol, two major risk factors for heart disease.

3. **Increased mental acuity** Memory loss can occur as a result of age, poor health, depression or medications. But unless there is irreversible brain damage, physical activity can invigorate and revitalize the mind. Aerobic exercise helps move blood and oxygen to all the body's organs, including the brain.

4. **Reduced risk of diabetes** Excess weight increases the risk of Type 2 or non-insulin-dependent diabetes mellitus (NIDDM). However, physically active people are less likely to develop this condition, and those who have NIDDM can reduce their blood sugar and their need for medication with more physical activity. Exercise increases the body's ability to use sugar for energy and thereby decreases the need for insulin.

   One study focused on the impact of exercise on the rate of NIDDM in 897 middle-aged Finnish men. Researchers adjusted their results for age, parental history of diabetes, alcohol consumption and other relevant factors and found men who engaged in more than 40 minutes per week of moderate exercise reduced their risk of NIDDM. This protective effect was more pronounced in men who were at high risk of developing diabetes, according to the study's authors.

5. **Pain relief** When you exercise, your body generates pain-killing endorphins. Moderate exercise also triggers the release of natural cortisone, which helps relieve the pain of osteoarthritis. Overweight people are more susceptible to osteoarthritis. Strength training, in particular, can decrease arthritis pain. It does not cure the condition, but stronger muscles may ease the strain and therefore the discomfort, according to a report from the National Institute on Aging.

6. **Increased bone density** Osteoporosis is a debilitating bone condition responsible for chronic pain, spine problems and bone fractures for millions of senior citizens, most of them women. In the United States, it afflicts 25 percent of the over-60 female population. In Canada, osteoporosis affects 25 percent of women over the age of 50, and 50 percent of women over 75. Bone loss is preventable and, to some extent, reversible. In one study, very sedentary 90-year-old nursing home residents performed mild exercises for 30 minutes, three times a week. On average, they experienced a 4.2 percent increase in their bone density.

7. **Longevity** Obese people face a higher rate of mortality. Exercise may help reduce that risk. One study focused on 40,417 post-menopausal women. Researchers found that, in general, the more frequent and intense their physical activity, the lower their risk of death from all causes.

8. **Increased strength** The National Institutes of Health found that men and women, between the ages of 86 and 96, tripled the muscular strength of their legs when they worked out with weights.

9. **Improved quality of sleep** One study investigated 43 individuals who were sedentary, free of cardiovascular disease and who reported some trouble sleeping. Part of the group underwent 16 weeks of moderately intense exercise (low-impact aerobics or walking), and the rest remained inactive. Those who exercised regularly experienced improvement in their quality of sleep.

10. **Improved energy level** Believe it or not, regular exercise can actually make you feel more energized and give you the vim and vigor to lead an active life.

Cellulite

Even with proper diet and exercise, many people, especially women, have a hard time getting rid of cellulite. In fact, more than 90 percent of women have cellulite. Cellulite is superficial fat that results from impaired circulation and enlargement of fat cells. Inactivity and poor circulation cause the connective tissue (fibrous tissue located below the skin) to pull on the skin and the fat cells to glob together, creating an "orange peel" appearance.

The unsightly appearance of cellulite sends many women panicking to the cosmetic counter for a magic cream or potion. Unfortunately, none of these products has been found to work. Losing excess body fat will make it less noticeable, yet even women of ideal body weight can suffer with cellulite. One technique that can be helpful in minimizing cellulite is a type of massage known as Endermologie®. This technique utilizes a machine of suction and rollers, which help increase circulation, improve fluid exchange and smooth the skin's surface. Benefits can be seen with as few as eight treatments. Therapeutic mud treatments, castor oil packs, Epsom salt baths and dry brushing are other strategies that can help improve circulation and improve cellulite.

STARTING YOUR WEIGHT-LOSS PROGRAM

It is one thing to know what it takes to lose weight and keep it off. It is another thing to actually implement it. Here are some suggestions:

- **Keep a food diary.** Before you decide what you need to change, take an objective look at what you are eating now. Donald D. Hensrud, M.D., a physician nutrition specialist at the Mayo Clinic, points out that most people underestimate the number of calories they eat by about 20 percent. "It's not intentional or devious," he states. "It's just that we're not good judges." Once you get an accurate look at what you are really eating, keep the nutrient-rich foods in your diet, and whittle down the fillers (refined carbohydrates, sweets, and snack foods).
- **Set manageable goals.** A 50-pound weight loss is daunting. Focus on five-pound increments instead. If you gradually lose one-half to one pound a week, you will lose five pounds in five to ten weeks. In the meantime, you will be shaking off some of your fattening habits and adopting healthier ones.
- **Make more daily health-promoting choices.** If you like to snack, choose fresh fruit over ice cream. Opt for low-fat sunflower seeds over high-fat potato chips. Order your mocha without whipped cream. Take the stairs instead of the elevator. Park your car farther away from your destination, so you do a little more walking. All of these small shifts in behavior add up to steady weight loss and improved overall health.

- **Take pride in your progress.** Modest losses can yield impressive health benefits. By losing ten pounds, you can lower your blood pressure significantly. When you lose ten excess kilograms, you: reduce your mortality by 20 to 25 percent; reduce angina symptoms by 91 percent; decrease total cholesterol by 10 percent; cut your risk of developing diabetes by more than 50 percent; and increase your exercise tolerance by 33 percent.
- **Make a commitment to lifelong changes.** Changing your diet and lifestyle for a month or two is a good start, but it is not enough. For long-term weight loss, you need to make long-term changes. Dr. Hensrud states, "I try to get [patients] to focus on the process rather than the end result.... They need to focus on making lasting lifestyle changes. The pounds will come off as a result."

HOW'S YOUR METABOLISM?

You have probably known (and possibly envied) a "fast metabolizer"—someone who eats two cheeseburgers, a large order of onion rings and a candy bar chaser for lunch. Then he complains that he has tried everything, but just cannot put on an ounce of weight.

It is obvious that we burn calories at different rates. Factors such as gender, age, diet, activity level, thyroid health, amount of sleep, amount of body fat, amount of muscle mass, body temperature, weight and genetics all influence our basal metabolic rate (BMR).

The "set point theory" refers to the amount of fat your body tries to maintain. This is the weight you maintain, give or take a few pounds—the weight you return to after an unsuccessful diet. Overweight people have a higher set point than their thinner counterparts. The challenge is to lower the set point.

The body works like a thermostat. If you have a high set point and you consume fewer calories, your body reacts as if you are starving. It lowers the rate at which you burn calories in a misguided attempt to conserve your set point of body fat. Due to your reduced BMR, it takes fewer calories to maintain the same weight. Dr. Conte states, "When we cut calories by going on a diet, the body cuts down on the number of calories burned after a few days of adaptation. This can ruin all our attempts to lose weight."

What determines our set point? One theory suggests that it is the number of fat cells we develop before birth, during infancy and during the adolescent growth phase. If we are overfed or overeat during these times, we may manufacture more fat cells.

If you have developed more fat cells during growth periods, such as infancy and adolescence, you are likely to have more body fat, a slower metabolism and a higher set point.

Naturally, this can be very frustrating for overweight people. Starvation diets lead to rebound weight gain, as the body tries desperately to hang on to its fat stores. As weight goes up and down, the set point gets higher and the BMR slows down.

The solution involves gradual dietary changes you can live with, consistent physical activity you can stick with and specific natural compounds that can help lower your set point and increase your BMR.

SUPPLEMENTS FOR WEIGHT LOSS

Diet and exercise are the cornerstones of healthy, long-term weight loss. However, certain natural compounds—in the context of reduced calorie intake and consistent physical activity—can be helpful in winning at weight loss. There are a variety of supplements on the market, which vary in their mechanism of action.

Finding the right supplement for your weight management strategies can:

• enhance your metabolism
• promote lean muscle mass
• prevent the storage of fat
• neutralize carbohydrates
• curb your appetite
• control sugar cravings.

While the shelves of pharmacies and health food stores are lined with weight-loss products, few are clinically tested for safety and efficacy. The following section outlines products that can help support healthy weight loss.

Cassia nomame

Cassia nomame is a member of the same plant family as cinnamon. Research has shown it to contain compounds that block the enzyme that digests fat. Fats that you ingest are absorbed into your system with the help of enzymes known as lipases. By blocking lipase activity, Cassia nomame is thought to reduce the amount of fat that gets into your body. While the research on casia nomame is quite preliminary, it is estimated to reduce the absorption of fat calories from a meal by about 30 percent.

In a 1997 issue of *Phytochemistry*, Japanese researchers reported that cassia nomame "showed a potent inhibitory effect on lipase." The study, using pancreatic lipase, showed a 28 percent inhibition of lipase activity.

In a more recent study published in the June 2000 edition of the *International Journal of Obesity* researchers showed that this lipase inhibitor is effective in preventing and ameliorating obesity, fatty liver and hypertriglyceridemia in rats fed a high-fat diet.

Cassia nomame may be a safer alternative to chitosan, another fat-inhibiting substance. Chitosan is a form of fiber, which binds with the fat in the stomach, thereby inhibiting digestion. Chitosan requires direct contact with fat in order to decrease the amount of fat calories absorbed and requires a relatively large dose. Cassia nomame works in much smaller amounts directly on the enzymes that breakdown the fats. As well, Chitosan has been found to have a negative effect on one's nutritional status by reducing the absorption of fat soluble vitamins, such as vitamins A, D, E and K. Side effects with chitosan have also been a problem, including gas, bloating and diarrhea.

Cassia nomame can be found in various weight loss supplements and formulas. The usual dosage is 150 mg of a 10:1 extract three times daily before meals.

Citrus aurantium (Advantra-Z)

Citrus aurantium is the immature dried fruit of the bitter orange. Citrus aurantium contains five adrenergic amines (chemicals that resemble adrenaline, especially in physiological action). These amines work together to provide thermogenic activity. Thermogenesis refers to an increase in the body's resting metabolic rate, so your body continues to burn more calories even when you are not working out. Citrus aurantium may also give your workouts more clout. By releasing free fatty acids during aerobic exercise, citrus aurantium can help provide more energy, thereby facilitating improved physical performance.

Citrus aurantium is thought to work by selectively stimulating beta-3 cell receptors in the body. Beta-3 receptors are located primarily in the fatty tissue and liver and stimulation of these receptors, activates lipolysis (fat breakdown) and thermogenesis, helping the body burn fat more efficiently.

Citrus aurantium versus Ephedra

Citrus aurantium is often compared to ephedra (ma huang), because it has a similar mechanism of action, but is better tolerated. Ephedra was previously a very popular supplement for weight loss because of its thermogenic properties—it boosts metabolism and also suppresses appetite. Both the FDA and Health Canada have banned the sale of supplements containing ephedra due to mounting evidence of side effects and health risks. The problem with ephedra is that it is not selective in its effects and is known to stimulate the central nervous system and drive the cardiovascular system to work harder. Use of ephedra, even at recommended dosages, has lead to increased heart rate and blood pressure, heart palpitations, muscle disturbances, dry mouth, nervousness, anxiety, seizures, stroke and even death!

Research on citrus aurantium

Researchers at McGill University's Nutrition and Food Science Center in Montreal explored the potential of Citrus aurantium. In their small study, researchers found that Citrus aurantium increased the thermogenic effect of food (TEF), meaning that the subjects burned more calories and stored less fat.

Researchers found a measurable increase in metabolic rate when Citrus aurantium was ingested. They state, "Furthermore, as no irregular changes in pulse pressure or blood pressure were reported, our results indicate that the alkaloid mixture is well-tolerated." Earlier studies also found that Citrus aurantium had comparable thermogenic effects to ephedra, but did not cause the side effects commonly associated with ephedra use.

Conjugated linoleic acid (CLA)

CLA is a derivative of linoleic acid, which is found naturally in certain foods, such as meat and dairy products. It has been found to offer a number of health benefits, including protection against cancer and atherosclerosis. As a weight loss aid, CLA has been shown to improve fat metabolism and maintain or improve lean muscle mass. Specifically it works by increasing lipolysis (fat breakdown) and enhancing fatty acid oxidation (promotes burning of fat).

The body does not manufacture CLA; therefore, we must get it through diet or supplements. Butter, whole milk, cheese and beef contain CLA. In fact, CLA was first isolated from hamburger in 1979. However, consuming large amounts of these foods is not recommended because of their high content of saturated fat.

As well, these foods don't provide as much CLA as they once did. Foods provide only a small amount of CLA—6.1 mg per gram of fat in butter and 4.3 mg per gram of fat in ground beef. Animals today are more likely to eat commercial feeds than grass, so their production of CLA is down significantly. Also, Americans have cut their consumption of meat and dairy products by about 50 percent. For these reasons supplements of CLA are recommended for those looking for the body fat reduction benefits.

Research on CLA

Several clinical studies published in peer-reviewed journals, have confirmed the effects of CLA for weight loss. The most widely studied CLA product on the market is Tonalin® CLA. Recently, a one year double-blind study was completed where the effects of Tonalin CLA were compared to placebo in 157 overweight adults. Researchers measured the participant's body fat mass and lean body mass. No changes were made to exercise or diet. At the end of the study it was found that a daily intake of 3.4g of Tonalin CLA produced an average 9 per cent reduction in body fat mass. There was also a small increase in lean body mass.

From this group 134 of the participants volunteered to participate in a continuation of this study to examine the long term safety of the product and to determine whether they could maintain their fat loss. The participants continued to take a dosage of 3.4 grams of Tonalin CLA per day for an additional 12 months. There were no serious adverse effects and it was found that indeed, the participants were able to maintain their initial fat loss.

A study published in *The Journal of Nutrition*, (Sept 2000) found that without a change in exercise or diet, participants taking CLA experienced an average reduction of six pounds of body fat, compared with a placebo group. In August 2001, a study that appeared in *The International Journal of Obesity* showed that male subjects classified as abdominally obese, lost an average of one inch from their waistlines in a four-week period when using CLA. Finally, a study published in *Lipids*, August 2001, found that of 53 patients, those taking CLA over the course of a 14-week trial experienced body fat reductions of 3.8 percent.

Some researchers feel that the current level of CLA in the typical North American diet is insufficient, and that supplementation may offer unique health benefits, particularly for weight loss. Research on CLA with regard to weight loss has found benefits at dosages of two to five grams daily. Most products on the market provide one gram CLA per capsule or softgel. CLA is very well tolerated and no side effects or drug interactions have been reported.

Green tea

Green tea is obtained from the herb *Camellia sinensis*. This popular beverage offers many health benefits. It has been shown to lower cholesterol and blood pressure, protect against certain cancers, block bacteria and viruses, improve digestion and reduce the risk of ulcers and strokes. Green tea has also been shown to support weight loss. It provides a source of caffeine (approx. 20 to 50 mg per cup), a known thermogenic agent. Green tea is also rich in catechins, a type of antioxidant. In preliminary research, the combination of these ingredients has been found to help promote weight loss by burning more fat calories. Researchers at the University of Geneva studied the effects of green tea on ten healthy young men, average age 25, who ranged from lean to mildly overweight. For six weeks, the men took two capsules at each meal: green tea extract plus 50 milligrams of caffeine; 50 milligrams of caffeine or a placebo.

The participants followed a routine weight maintenance diet. Three times during the study, they spent 24 hours in a special room where the investigators measured their respiration and energy expenditure. Energy expenditures (the number of calories used during a 24-hour period) were 4 percent higher for men taking green tea extract compared to those taking caffeine or placebo. They also found evidence that men taking the green tea extract used more fat calories than those taking the placebo.

There was no difference between the caffeine users and the placebo users in terms of either overall calorie burning or fat calorie burning. The researchers concluded that the benefits seen in the green tea group cannot be explained by caffeine intake alone. They suggested that the caffeine interacted with natural substances in green tea, called flavonoids, to alter the body's use of norepinephrine, a chemical transmitter in the nervous system and increase the rate of calorie burning. Unlike some weight loss products, green tea does not contain high amounts of caffeine, and it did not affect the heart rate in the study participants.

In 2002, researchers at the National Institute of Health and Medical Research in Marseille, France reported the results of a study of a green tea extract in 70 moderately obese adults (90 percent women) ranging in age from 20–69 years. The patients took a standardized green tea extract in capsules providing 375 milligrams of green tea catechins per day for three months. Over the course of the study, both the waist measurement and body weight of the patients steadily declined. In the end, the decrease in body weight averaged 4.6 percent and waist circumference had decreased by an average of 4.48 percent.

For those who enjoy drinking green tea, studies have found health benefits with ranges between three and ten cups or more daily. Green tea can also be taken in capsule or tablet form. The usual recommended dosage is one tablet/capsule three to four times daily of a product that provides 90 milligrams of EGCG and 50 milligrams of caffeine per dosage. Although green tea is well tolerated, it should be used cautiously by those sensitive to caffeine, such as those with high blood pressure, kidney disease, insomnia or increased intraocular (eye) pressure.

Hydroxycitric acid

Hydroxycitric acid (HCA) is a compound derived from the fruit Garcinia cambogia, which is native to South and Southeast Asia. HCA has been popular as a weight loss supplement for years. It appears that HCA supports weight loss by reducing appetite and inhibiting fat storage without affecting the central nervous system. There may be other benefits as well, as newer research has found that it can reduce cholesterol and triglycerides.

There has been some controversy surrounding the benefits of HCA for weight loss. Early clinical studies found mixed results. In reviewing this research it appears that this may be due to poor study design and differences in potency and quality of the products tested. Newer research on HCA has used a more potent formulation and achieved better results.

One of the most comprehensive studies on HCA was recently conducted by researchers at Georgetown University Medical Center (Washington, DC) in conjunction with Andhra University (India). This study involved 83 moderately overweight individuals who were randomized to receive one of the following three treatments over an eight-week period:

- Super CitriMax® 4667 mg (60 percent extract delivering 2800 mg HCA)
- Super CitriMax® Formula: Super CitriMax 4667 mg (60 percent extract providing 2800 mg HCA), ChromeMate 4 mg providing 400 mcg elemental chromium and Gymnema sylvestre extract 400 mg providing 100 mg gymnemic acid.
- Placebo

Subjects were provided with meals that delivered 2,000 kcal per day and underwent a 30-minute walking exercise program five days a week, which was supervised by a trained exercise specialist.

Changes in body weight, lipid profile (triglycerides, LDL, HDL and total cholesterol), serum serotonin levels (a mechanism of appetite control and eating behavior), Body Mass Index, fat metabolites and appetite control (food consumption) were assessed.

Results of this study found that both the Super CitriMax and the Super CitriMax Formula significantly:

• curb appetite and reduce food intake
• inhibit fat synthesis and increases fat "burning"
• reduce body weight and decreases Body Mass Index (an indicator of healthy body weight)
• reduce cholesterol levels.

No serious side effects have been reported with HCA. While earlier studies found benefits in dosages around 1200 to 1500 milligrams HCA daily, the new research supports greater benefits at a higher dosage, such as 2800 milligrams per day.

NeOpuntia®

NeOpuntia is a patented, fat-blocking ingredient developed by Laboratoires BIO SERAE (France). It is manufactured from dehydrated leaves of a cactus called *Opuntia ficus-indica*. NeOpuntia reduces the amount of fat absorbed in response to a fatty meal. Specifically it irreversibly binds to excess fat in the gastrointestinal tract, and prevents it from being broken down into smaller units that could pass through the intestinal wall.

According to researchers, the fat binding properties of NeOpuntia result from its high content of dietary fibers (>45%), called NeOfiber and NeOmicel. NeOfiber is a non-water-soluble dietary fiber complex. NeOfiber absorbs fat by hydrophobic interaction. NeOmicel is a soluble dietary fiber complex that works by creating a fluid gel, which stabilizes the primary hydrophobic interactions with dietary fats. Together these fibers prevent the break down and absorption of dietary fats. Other components of NeOpuntia include soluble sugars, proteins, lipids, minerals (calcium, potassium and magnesium), vitamins (b-carotene, vitamin C), and amino acids.

A double-blind, cross-over pilot study was conducted on a group of 10 individuals to test the fat binding capacity of NeOpuntia. Subjects were given either 1.6 grams of NeOpuntia or placebo with each meal, followed by a one week washout period. Subjects were then crossed over and retested. A strict diet was followed to ensure standardized lipid intake. Researchers measured fat excretion and found that NeOpuntia increased the rate of lipids excreted by 27.4% in comparison to placebo. No side effects were noted. In another study 30 subjects given 1200 mg NeOpuntia per day (as part of a multi-ingredient formulation) vs. placebo for 30 days. Average body weight was reduced from 78.5 to 73.4 kg in those given NeOpuntia. New studies are underway to further validate the benefits of NeOpuntia.

The recommended dosage of NeOpuntia is 1-2 g taken 30 minutes to 1 hour after each meal. Various products are available on the market including tablets and capsules.

Phase 2®

Phase 2 is a standardized extract derived from the white kidney bean that promotes weight loss by neutralizing ingested starches. Foods high in starch include bread, pasta, rice, potatoes and baked goods—all the foods we love and tend to over-indulge in. In clinical studies, Phase 2 has been shown to reduce the amount of starch absorbed from starchy meals and promote loss of body fat.

Phase 2 works in the intestine by temporarily inhibiting the activity of alpha amylase, the enzyme that breaks down starch into smaller glucose (sugar) molecules. As a result, fewer starch calories are absorbed from a meal.

Research on Phase 2

Several studies have been undertaken to examine the weight loss benefits of Phase 2. In an in-vitro test, Phase 2 neutralized 2,250 starch calories, or the equivalent of over one pound of spaghetti or one loaf of bread. In one study, ten subjects were given a standardized meal containing 60 grams of starch (four slices of white bread) and either placebo or 1500 grams of Phase 2. Postprandial (after meal) blood sugar levels were measured as an index of starch absorption. Participants went about their regular work activity and blood sugar was measured every 30 minutes for four hours. Starch absorption averaged 57 percent less in those given Phase 2.

Participants receiving Phase 2 in a second study averaged an 85 percent reduction in plasma glucose response. This study was identical in design to the first, with the exception that test subjects were inactive during the course of the study, with plasma glucose measurements being taken every 15 minutes for the first hour, and every 20 minutes for the second hour. This study was undertaken to determine whether differences in physical activity could influence the results. The results of these two studies strongly indicate that a significant portion of the starch calories from the test meal were undigested when taken along with Phase 2. Participants given Phase 2 reported no adverse side effects in either study.

A more extensive double-blind placebo-controlled study looked at the effects of Phase 2 in 60 overweight individuals aged 25–45. Volunteers were selected based on a stable body weight, ranging from 5 to 15 kilograms or 12 to 33 pounds over optimal body weight, for 30 days prior to participation in the study. They were instructed to follow a recommended diet with daily consumption of starchy foods during one of the principal meals. Participants consuming 500 milligrams of Phase 2 once daily before one of the principal meals lost an average of 6.45 pounds (3.96 percent of their body weight) by the end of the 30-day study, whereas those consuming a placebo lost an average of 0.76 pounds (0.47 percent of their body weight). In addition, those on Phase 2 lost 10.45 percent of fat body mass, 3.44 percent waist circumference, 1.44 percent thigh circumference and 1.39 percent hip circumference. These losses occurred without any change in lean muscle mass. Placebo participants had much smaller losses of 1.3 percent, 0.53 percent, 0.39 percent and 0.10 percent respectively.

The most recent study on Phase 2 was conducted at Northridge Hospital Medical Center, UCLA. It was found that those given Phase 2 lost an average of four pounds in eight weeks, and experienced an average 26-point reduction in triglycerides and greater energy. In comparison, those given placebo lost only 1.6 pounds. This study was published recently in *Alternative Medicine Review.*

New research on Phase 2 is currently underway in New York and California to evaluate the possible benefits for this supplement in aiding with weight loss among adolescents. Due to its clean safety profile, researchers feel that it represents a promising new approach to managing adolescent obesity, a growing epidemic among our youth.

This carbohydrate neutralizing effect represents a novel approach to weight loss and may be particularly helpful for those struggling with both obesity and diabetes. Phase 2 is safe and well tolerated and is not known to interact with any drugs or supplements. The recommended dosage of Phase 2 is 500 to 1500 milligrams before starchy meals. Phase 2 is available in a variety of forms including tablets, capsules and soft chews.

Satise®

Portion control is a critical part of a successful weight loss program, but cutting down on food intake is sometimes easier said than done. Those with a hearty appetite often don't feel satisfied with smaller portions and this can lead to temptation and binge eating. The key to managing hunger and appetite is to make small gradual changes to your diet. Eating small frequent meals with nutrient-dense, high-fiber, low-calorie foods can help to control appetite. For those requiring a little extra help, there is a new supplement available that works naturally to manage appetite called Satise.

The active ingredient in Satise is a protein extract derived from potatoes called Proteinase Inhibitor II. This supplement works in the intestine to signal the release of a naturally occurring compound called cholecystokinin (CCK). CCK is one of the key hormones involved in hunger control. It is normally released into the blood after a meal and it acts on the stomach to slow emptying, which helps to make you feel full. CCK also acts on the brain to trigger feelings of satiety (satisfaction).

Clinical studies have shown that Satise significantly elevates CCK levels, which promotes a feeling of fullness thus reducing food intake. At the North American Association for the Study of Obesity, researchers reported that hunger ratings were reduced by 30% after taking Satise. In other studies, Satise was found to reduce blood sugar levels after a meal and promote weight loss.

Unlike other appetite suppressants, Satise does not contain any stimulants, so it won't affect blood pressure or heart rate. In fact, there aren't any serious side effects with this product. Although this supplement is extracted from potatoes, it does not contain any carbohydrates and provides less than four calories per capsule. The recommended dosage is one capsule 60 minutes before the two largest meals of the day.

WEIGHT-LOSS DRUGS: Buyer Beware

Always beware of products that make outrageous claims. If it sounds too good to be true, it usually is. When choosing a product, consult with your pharmacist or health care provider for assistance. Important questions to ask are:

1. Has the product been clinically tested?

2. Are there any side effects or interactions?

3. How should the product be taken (before meals, with food)?

4. How long can I take this product?

Prescription drugs

Drugs are occasionally prescribed for people with a BMI over 30, or people with a BMI over 27 who also have other risk factors or diseases. Typically, these drugs are used to complement dietary therapy and physical activity, and should never be taken in place of lifestyle strategies. There are two main categories of weight-loss medications:

- Appetite suppressants decrease appetite and increase the feeling of being full. Side effects include nervousness, insomnia and irritability, increased blood pressure, nausea, diarrhea and dry mouth.
- Drugs affecting the gastrointestinal tract, such as orlistat, decrease the amount of dietary fat that the body absorbs. Reported side effects include loose bowel movements, abdominal cramps and nausea.

DO YOU REALLY NEED TO LOSE WEIGHT?

Certainly, obesity is a profound medical problem facing North American society. People with excess body fat need to slim down for better heart health, a lower risk of certain cancers and diabetes, fewer symptoms of osteoarthritis and a host of other health benefits.

However, the other extreme is just as dangerous. An estimated 1 percent of American females suffer from anorexia nervosa, a potentially life-threatening illness characterized by excessive dieting and weight loss. Anorexics are typically perfectionists, have busy and uninvolved parents, and suffer from severe depression. Too much weight loss can increase the risk of osteoporosis in later years and can damage the heart and other organs.

In the United States, an estimated 2 percent of college students and 1 percent of women in general suffer from bulimia nervosa. People who suffer from bulimia are likely to binge on food, then force themselves to vomit. They may also take laxatives and diuretics to compensate for their bingeing. Bulimics may or may not be overweight, are usually female, are often older teens or young adults, and are likely to bottle up anger because they cannot express emotions in a healthy, constructive way. Bulimia is associated with health problems such as tears in the stomach lining, ruptures, irregular heartbeat, kidney damage from potassium deficiency, damaged tooth enamel and cessation of menstrual periods.

Although 90 to 95 percent of people with eating disorders are women, these conditions occasionally affect men, too. The factors that predispose men to eating disorders are similar to those that affect women:

• History of being overweight or dieting
• Involvement in activities where thinness is important, such as running, track and field, horseback riding, wrestling and body building

- Involvement in careers that value thinness, such as modeling and acting
- Living among people who equate thinness with attractiveness

Who has an "ideal" body?

Considering the slim images that bombard us from television, movies and magazines, it is no wonder people—especially young women—feel fat even though they are not. The typical model is between 5 feet 8 inches and 5 feet 10 inches tall and weighs 120 pounds. While her knee joints are wider than her thighs, her skinny frame is what most women seek. In contrast, the average North American woman is 5 feet 4 inches tall and weighs 138 pounds. Approximately one out of 40,000 women has a "model-perfect" body. Clearly, this is an unrealistic and possibly unhealthy ideal for the vast majority of women. Interestingly, Marilyn Monroe, the pinup girl for the 1950s, wore a size 14. Very few people objected to her appearance.

FINDING A HEALTHY BALANCE

Being either too fat or too thin creates health problems. Obesity is by far the greatest health dilemma in North American society, but it is important not to go overboard in the other direction.

For example, if you are a 5-foot, 10-inch man and you weigh 165 pounds, your BMI is 24—within normal range. You may not fit into the jeans you wore in high school, but you probably do not need to lose weight. Keep eating right, exercise consistently and make sure your BMI stays under 25.

If you are a 5-foot, 4-inch woman and you weigh 135 pounds, your BMI is 23, which is fine. You may not resemble super model Kate Moss, but you can stand your ground in a strong wind.

For middle-aged women, gaining a few pounds may have a

protective function. One theory is that women tend to gain some weight around menopause because their bodies are trying to hang on to estrogen, which is stored in fat tissue. A 45-year-old woman should not expect to have the same figure she had when she was 16, but she also needs to stay within a healthy BMI. If her weight is too low, she may increase her risk of osteoporosis; if her weight is too high, she becomes more susceptible to diabetes, heart disease, stroke and certain cancers.

To reach and maintain a healthy weight, learn to make critical distinctions between weight loss and fat loss, between diet and nutrition, and between being thin and being healthy. Clearly, for long-term success, you need to emphasize fat loss, nutrition and being healthy.

TAKE IT SLOWLY

You have heard it before, and it is true: "you didn't put the weight on overnight, and you're not going to take it off overnight." Health authorities, including The Mayo Clinic, recommend losing one pound a week if you are a woman; two pounds a week if you are a man. (Because of their higher metabolic rate, it is easier for men to lose weight more quickly.)

If you lose one pound of body fat a week, you will lose 52 pounds in a year. You may feel as though you are spinning your wheels, but the slow, gradual progress is the kind that sticks. The right supplementation can help you stay on track as you develop healthier eating habits and become more physically active.

If you backslide once in a while, don't despair—it is not all or nothing. Every little bit helps. Change a little and get less results; change a lot and the difference in how you feel will be dramatic.

SEVEN-DAY HEALTHY MEAL PLAN FOR SAFE AND SUCCESSFUL WEIGHT LOSS

	MONDAY (Day 1)	TUESDAY (Day 2)	WEDNESDAY (Day 3)
BREAKFAST	– Power Shake: 1-2 scoops Protein Powder.*** Add 350 mL (8 oz) water, milk or soy milk and shake well. May also be combined with berries, bananas or other fruit in blender with ice.	– Power Shake – 30 g almonds – 500 mL water	– Power Shake – 250 mL fruit salad – 500 mL water
SNACK	– Handful of grapes or an apple – Herbal or green tea	– Energy Bar** – Herbal or green tea	– 175 mL 1% MF yogurt – Herbal or green tea
LUNCH	– Sandwich: 60–120 g chicken*, 2 slices multi-grain bread, 1 tsp. mustard, sliced tomato and lettuce – 175 mL 1% MF yogurt – 500 mL water	– 2 cups Green Salad – 1/2–1 can (4 oz) water packed tuna* drained, – 25 mL salad dressing – 1/2 whole wheat pita – 500 mL water	– Veggie Wrap: 1–8-inch soft whole-wheat tortilla, sliced tomato, cucumber, green pepper, onion – 50 mL hummus – 1 medium apple – 500 mL water
SNACK	– 50 g trail mix – 500 mL water	– 1 orange – 500 mL water	– 1 pear – 500 mL water
DINNER	– 100–150g* baked fish – 125 mL steamed brown rice – 125 mL green beans – 125 mL carrots – 500 mL water	– 100–150g* chicken – 1/2 small sweet potato, baked – 250 mL cooked broccoli – 500 mL water	– 100–150g* pork tenderloin – 125 mL steamed brown rice – 250 mL stir-fried green vegetables – 500 mL water

1 oz = 30 g or mL

* Men can choose larger serving size.
** Refer to Table 3 for a list of recommended energy bars.
*** Refer to Table 4 for recommended Protein Powders

THURSDAY (Day 4)	FRIDAY (Day 5)	SATURDAY (Day 6)	SUNDAY (Day 7)
– Power Shake – 1 medium orange – 500 mL water	– Power Shake – 175 mL 1% MF yogurt - top with 30 g dried fruit and nuts – 500 mL water	– 2 poached eggs with 1 slice whole grain toast – 500 mL water	– 250 mL cooked oatmeal – Top with 30-60 mL flaxseed, sliced apple and cinnamon – 500 mL water
– Energy Bar** – Herbal or green tea	– 125 mL sliced peaches – 50 mL 1% cottage cheese – Herbal or green lea	– 175 mL 1% MF yogurt – Herbal or green tea	– 50 mL almonds – 500 mL water
– 175 mL mixed bean salad – 1 tomato, sliced – 25 mL salad dressing – 1/2 whole wheat pita – 500 mL water	– 250 mL Vegetable Soup – 1/2 whole-wheat pita – 1/2–1 can* salmon, drained – 25 mL light mayo or yogurt – 500 mL water	– 250 mL bean or lentil soup – 1/2–1 sandwich*: 60–120 g turkey, lettuce, sliced tomato, mustard – 250 mL skim or 1% milk	– Chef's Salad: 500 mL greens, sliced raw vegetables, 1 hard-boiled egg, 1/2 can 2oz water-packed tuna, 50 mL chickpeas, 25 mL salad dressing – 175 mL 1% MF yogurt
– 50 g trail mix – 500 mL water	– 2 plums – 500 mL water	– 1 apple – 500 mL water	– 125 mL sliced peaches – 500 mL water
– 2-Egg Omelet: bell peppers, mushrooms, 25g feta cheese, 30 mL salsa – 1 slice whole grain bread – Tossed green salad – 25 mL salad dressing – 500 mL water	– Chicken Spinach Salad: 2 cups raw spinach, sliced mushrooms, bean sprouts, sliced strawberries, 100–150g* grilled chicken, – 25 mL Japanese dressing (Soy sauce mixed with vinegar and olive oil, seasoning to taste – 1 small whole grain roll – 500 mL water	– 250–375mL* vegetable or whole wheat pasta cooked al denté, 100-150 g Tomato sauce with lean ground meat – Green salad, 25 mL salad dressing – 500 mL water	–Turkey Tacos: 1–2* 8–inch, soft whole wheat tortillas with ground turkey, seasonings, chopped veggies as desired, grated part skim cheese and salsa – 500 mL water

TABLE 1   GLYCEMIC INDEX

Preferred	Moderate Use	Minimize
Low Glycemic Foods (GI < 55)	**Moderate Glycemic Foods (GI 55–70)**	**High Glycemic Foods (GI>70)**
Almonds	Bran cereal	Bagel
Apple	Bread, whole wheat	Bananas
Apricots, dried	Buckwheat	Bread, white
Barley	Cantaloupe	Candy (sugar)
Broccoli	Carrots	Corn chips
Bulgar	Corn	Corn flakes
Cherries	Grapes	Couscous
Chickpeas	Honey	Dates, dried
Grapefruit	Oatmeal	Doughnuts
Kidney beans	Peas	Graham crackers
Lentils	Pineapple	Ice cream
Milk	Pita bread	Kaiser roll
Oranges	Popcorn	Mango
Pasta, whole wheat	Raisins	Potato (baked)
Pears	Rice (brown and basmati)	Pretzel
Plums	Rye bread	Rice, short grain white
Rice bran	Sourdough bread	Rice Cakes
Rice, wild	Sweet potato (yams)	Soda crackers
Soy beans	Sucrose (table sugar)	Soft drinks
Yogurt	Whole wheat bread	Watermelon

The glycemic index (GI) ranks carbohydrates based on their impact on blood sugar levels. It compares foods to glucose which is assigned a value of 100. To determine the GI, scientists measure blood sugar after a test food supplying 50 grams of carbohydrate. Carbohydrates that are broken down quickly cause a fast and high increase in blood sugar and therefore have a higher GI.

Following a low GI diet causes a lower rise in blood sugar levels after a meal and this offers a number of health benefits: supports weight loss by keeping you feeling full longer, prolongs physical endurance, improves the body's sensitivity to insulin and improves diabetic control.

For further information on the glycemic index, visit the University of Sydney's website: www.glycemicindex.com

TABLE 2 BODY MASS INDEX

BMI (kg/m2)	19	20	21	22	23	24	25	26	27	28	29	30	35	40
Height (inches)	Weight in pounds													
58	91	96	100	105	110	115	119	124	129	134	138	143	167	191
59	94	99	104	109	114	119	124	128	133	138	143	148	173	198
60	97	102	107	112	118	123	128	133	138	143	148	153	179	204
61	100	106	111	116	122	127	132	137	143	148	153	158	185	211
62	104	109	115	120	126	131	136	142	147	153	158	164	191	218
63	107	113	118	124	130	135	141	146	152	158	163	169	197	225
64	110	116	122	128	134	140	145	151	157	163	169	174	204	232
65	114	120	126	132	138	144	150	156	162	168	174	180	210	240
66	118	124	130	136	142	148	155	161	167	173	179	186	216	247
67	121	127	134	140	146	153	159	166	172	178	185	191	223	255
68	125	131	138	144	151	158	164	171	177	184	190	197	230	262
69	128	135	142	149	155	162	169	176	182	189	196	203	236	270
70	132	139	146	153	160	167	174	181	188	195	202	207	243	278
71	136	143	150	157	165	172	179	186	193	200	208	215	250	286
72	140	147	154	162	169	177	184	191	199	206	213	221	258	294
73	144	151	159	166	174	182	189	197	204	212	219	227	265	302
74	148	155	163	171	179	186	194	202	210	218	225	233	272	311
75	152	160	168	176	184	192	200	208	216	224	232	240	279	319
76	156	164	172	180	189	197	205	213	221	230	238	246	287	328

Table 3 Recommended Energy Bars

Balance®	Slim Down™
Genisoy®	Luna™ Bar

TABLE 4 RECOMMENDED PROTEIN SUPPLEMENTS

Trans-Plex™ Natural Meal Replacement by Natural-Edge
Fat Wars Ultimate Protein™ by Preferred Nutrition
Proteins+™ by Genuine Health
Jarrow Formulas® Whey Protein

RECOMMENDED FIBER SUPPLEMENTS
Milled Flaxseed
- A nutty tasting meal that provides a good source of dietary fiber, omega-3 fatty acids and lignans
- Provides 3.9 grams dietary fiber per 2 tablespoons
- Recommended use: 2 tablespoons daily mixed with juice, water or yogurt

Complete Sweet™ by Natural-Edge
- A sweet tasting, fiber supplement that provides 3 grams of soluble fiber per teaspoon and Xylitol (a natural ingredient that has been shown to prevent dental cavities).

Satisfibre+ by Genuine Health
- This great tasting fibre powder provides 10 grams total dietary fiber per serving and is low glycemic. It contains a mix of both soluble and insoluble fibers from oats, fructo-oligosaccharides, flax seeds and fruits providing 10 grams fiber per serving.

FibreLean™
- A proprietary blend of soluble and insoluble fibers from organic fruit and vegetable fibers providing 10 grams total fiber per serving.

PGX™ by Natural Factors
- A blend of soluble fibers that can absorb more than 600 times their weight in water. This product is available in both capsule and powder form.

Please note: Good food sources of fiber include raw fruits and vegetables, whole grains, beans, legumes, nuts and seeds.

HELPFUL RESOURCES AND PRODUCT LINKS
For general information on herbs, vitamins and nutritional supplements:

- www.healthwell.com
- www.pdrhealth.com
- www.wholehealthmd.com

For information on the products discussed in this booklet:

- Fat Wars Ultimate Protein™: www.fatwars.com
- Phase 2® Starch Neutralizer: www.phase2info.com
- Super Citrimax: www.InterHealthUSA.com
- Tonalin® CLA: www.tonalin.com
- Trans-Plex Natural Fat Burner MRP: www.natural-edge.com
- NeOpuntia® Fat Blocker: www.neopuntia.com
- PGX™: www.slimstyles.com

OTHER HEALTH LINKS
- Author's website: wwwsherrytorkos.com
- American College of Sports Medicine: http://acsm.org/index.asp
- American Heart Association Fitness Resource: www.just-move.org
- Centers for Disease Control and Prevention: www.cdc.gov
- The Mayo Clinic: www.mayoclinic.com
- The National Women's Health Information Center: www.4woman.gov
- National Institutes of Health: www.nih.gov
- Reuters Health (for the latest medical and healthcare news): www.reutershealth.com
- Web MD: www.webmd.com

Adlercreutz H, et al. Inhibition of human aromotase by mammalian lignans and isoflavonoid phytroestrogens. J Steroid Biochem Molec Biol 1993, 44(2):147–151.

American Institute of Preventive Medicine: Eating disorders (anorexia and bulimia). Medical Self-Care, Healthworld Online, 1996.

Ballerini, R. Evaluation of efficacy and safety of a food supplement for weight control through the reduced calories-intake from carbohydrates vs. placebo. Data on file. Pharmachem Laboratories, Kearny, New Jersey, 2002.

Belury, M., et al. Protection against cancer and heart disease by the dietary fatty acid, conjugated linoleic acid: potential mechanisms of action. *Nutrition & Diseases Update Journal* 1997, 1(2).

Birmingham CL, Muller JL, Palepn A, Spinelli JJ, Anise AH: Cost of obesity in Canada. CMAJ1999, 160: 483–488.

Blankson, H., Stakkestad, J.A., Fagertun, H., et al. Conjugated linoleic acid reduces body fat mass in overweight and obese humans. J Nutr. 2000 Dec, 130(12): 2943–8.

Brehm, B.J., Seeley, R.J., Daniels, S.R., et al. "A Randomized Trial Comparing a Very Low Carbohydrate Diet and a Calorie-Restricted Low Fat Diet on Body Weight and Cardiovascular Risk Factors in Healthy Women," *The Journal of Clinical Endocrinology and Metabolism*, 88(4), 2003, pp. 1617–1623.

Carmona, Richard H. M.D., M.P.H., F.A.C.S., Surgeon General, U.S. Public Health Service, U.S. Department of Health and Human Services. Statements made before the Subcommittee on Competition, Infrastructure, and Foreign Commerce Committee on Commerce, Science, and Transportation United States Senate, released March 2, 2004.

Chantre P, Lairon D. Recent findings of green tea extract AR25 (Exolise) and its activity for the treatment of obesity. *Phytomedicine* 2002, 9: 3–8.

Colker, C.M., et al. Effects of Citrus aurantium extract, caffeine, and St. John's wort on body fat loss, lipid levels, and mood states in overweight healthy adults. *Curr Ther Res* 1999, 60: 145–153.

Dansinger, M.L., Gleason, J. L., Griffith, J.L., et al., "One Year Effectiveness of the Atkins, Ornish, Weight Watchers, and Zone Diets in Decreasing Body Weight and Heart Disease Risk." Presented at the American Heart Association Scientific Sessions November 12, 2003 in Orlando, Florida.

DeLany, J.P., Blohm, E., Truett, A.A., Scimeca, J.A., West, D.B. Conjugated linoleic acid rapidly reduces body fat content in mice without affecting energy intake. *Am J Physiol* 1999, 276 (4 Pt 2): R 1172R 1179.

Dulloo, A.G., et al. The thermogenic properties of ephedrine/methylxantine mixtures 11: human studies. *IntJ Obes* 1986, 10: 467–481.

Dulloo, A.G., Duret, C., Rohrer, D., et al. Efficacy of a green tea extract rich in catechin polyphenols and caffeine in increasing 24-h energy expenditure and fat oxidation in humans. *Am J Clin Nutr* 1999; 70: 1040–5.

Foster, G.D., Wyatt, H.R., Hill, J.O., et al., "A Randomized Trial of a Low-Carbohydrate Diet for Obesity," The New England Journal of Medicine, 348 (21), 2003, pp. 2082–2090.

Gaullier JM, Halse J, Høye K, et al. Conjugated linoleic acid supplementation for 1 y reduces body fat mass in healthy overweight humans. *Am J Clin Nutr* 2004; 79:1118 –25

Health Canada. 1990 National Population Health Survey, Canadian Community Health Survey 2000/2001.

Hoffstedt, J., et al. The metabolic syndrome is related to B3-adrenoceptor receptivity in visceral adipose tissue. *Diabetologia* 1996, 39: 383–844

Kandulska, K., Nogowski, L., Szkudelski, T. Effect of some phytoestrogens on metabolism of rat adipocytes. *Reprod Nutr Dev* 1999, 39: 497–501.

King A.C., et al. Moderate-intensity exercise and self-rated quality of sleep in older adults: a randomized controlled trial. *Journal of the American Medical Association* 1997, 277: 32–37.

King, B.J., *Fat Wars*. Toronto: John Wiley & Sons Canada, Ltd., 2000.

Kramer F.M., et al. Long-term follow-up of behavioural treatment of obesity: Patterns of regain among men and women. *Intl J Obesiy* 1989; 13: 123–126.

Kushi L.H., et al. Physical activity and mortality in postmenopausal women. 1997; 277: 1287–1292.

Lean ME, et al. Waist Circumference as a measure for indicating need for weight management. *BMJ* 1995; 311:158-161.

Lynch J, et al: Moderately intense physical activities and high levels of cardiorespiratory fitness reduce the risk of non-insulin-dependent diabetes mellitus in middle-aged men. *Arch Intern Med* 1996; 156:1307-1314.

MacDonald HB. Conjugated linoleic acid and disease prevention: a review of current knowledge. *Journal of the Amer-Coll of Nutrition* 2000; 19(2):111S-118S.

Manson JE, et al. Body Weight and Mortality. *N Engl J Med* 1995; 333:677-85.

Mokdad AH, Bowman BA, Ford ES, Vinicor F, Marks JS, Koplan JP. The continuing epidemics of obesity and diabetes in the United States., IAMA 2001; 286(10):1195-2000.

National Institute of Diabetes and Digestive and Kidney Diseases. Understanding Adult Obesity. NIH Publ. No. 94-3680. Rockville, MD: National Institutes of Health, 1993.

National Institutes of Health. Consensus conference on methods for voluntary weight loss and control. *Ann Int Med* 1992; 116:942-49.

Office of the Surgeon General, "Overweight and Obesity: The Surgeon General's Call To Action To Prevent and Decrease Overweight and Obesity", December, 2001. Accessed September 3, 2002. Available online at: http://www.surgeon-general.gov/topics/obesity

Park Y, Albright KJ, Storkson JM, Liu W, Cook ME, Pariza MW: Changes in body composition in mice during feeding and withdrawal of conjugated linoleic acid. *Lipids* 1998; 34(3):243-248.

Park Y, et al: Effect of conjugated linoleic acid on body composition in mice. *Lipids* 1997; 32(8):853-858.

Passwater RA: America's no. 1 health problem: overweight but undernourished. Interviews with Nutritional Experts. HealthWorld Online, July 13, 1999.

64 | References

Pi-Sunyer FX, et al: Medical hazards of obesity. *Ann Intern Med* 1993; 119:655-660.

Preuss, H.G., Bagchi, D., Bagchi, M., Rao, C.V.S., Satyanarayana, S., Dey. D.K., Efficacy of a Novel, Natural Extract of (–)Hydroxycitric Acid(HCA-SX) and a Combination of HCA-SX, Niacin-Bound Chromium and *Gymnema sylvestre* Extract in Weight Management in Human Volunteers: A Pilot Study, *Nutrition Research*, 24: 45–58, 2004.

Preuss, H.G., Bagchi, D., Bagchi, M., Rao, C.V.S., Dey, D.K. and Satyanarayana, S., Effects of a Natural Extract of (–)Hydroxycitric Acid(HCA-SX) and a Combination of HCA-SX plus Niacin-Bound Chromium and *Gymnema sylvestre* Extract on Weight Loss, *Diabetes, Obesity and Metabolism*, 6: 171–180, 2004.

Quillin P: Controlling food binges: correcting nutritional imbalances to tame the appetite. *Nature's Impact* February/March 1998, 46-49.

Report of the Task Force on the Treatment of Obesity. Ottawa, ON: Minister of Supplies and Services Canada, 1991.

Riserus, U, Berlund L, Vessby B. Conjugated linoleic acid (CLA) reduced abdominal adipose tissue in obese middle-aged men with signs of the metabolic syndrome: a randomised controlled trial. *Int J Obes Rekzt Metah Disord* 2001 Aug; 25(8):1129-35.

Scandinavian Clinical Research AS, Kjeller, Norway. *The Journal of International Medical Research* 2001; 29:392-296.

Shimizu K, Ozeki M, Iino A, Nakajyo S, Urakawa N, Atsuchi M. Structure-activity relationships of triterpenoid derivatives -extracted from Gymnema inodorurn leaves on glucose absorption. Jprz, I Phczrmczcol. 2001; 86(2):223-9.

Shrier I. Stretching before exercise: an evidence based approach. *Br J Sports Med* 2000 Oct; 34(5):324-5.

Smedman A, Vessby B. Conjugated linoleic acid supplementation in humans—metabolic effects. *Lipids*. 2001 Aug; 36(8):773-81.

Thom E: A pilot study with the aim of studying the efficacy and tolerability of Tonalin CLA on the body composition in humans. Medstat Research, Ltd., of Lillestrom, Norway, 1997.

U.S. Congress, House. *Deception and Fraud in the Diet Industry. Part 1.* Washington, DC: Government Printing Office, 101st Congress, 2nd Session, 1990, pp101-150.

Vigilante K, Flynn M: *Low-Fat Lies, High-Fat Frauds.* LifeLine Press, 1999.

World Health Organization. *Obesity: Preventing and Managing the Global Epidemic. Report of a WHO Consultation on Obesity.* Geneva: WHO, 1998.

Yamamoto M, Shimura S, Itoh Y, Ohsaka T, Egawa M, Inoue S. Anti-obesity effects of lipase inhibitor CT-I1, an extract from edible herbs, Nomame Herba, on rats fed a high-fat diet. *Int J Ohes Relat Metah Di.sord*. 2000; 24(6):758-64.

Yarnasaki M, Mansho K, Mishima H, Kasai 1V1, Sugano M, Tachibana H, Yamada K: Dietary effect of conjugated linoleic acid on lipid levels in white adipose tissue of Spraque-Dawley rats. *l3iosci Biotechnoll3iochem* 1999; 63(6):1104-1106.

Zimmerman M: Avoiding fat-free rebound. *Nature's Impact* December/January 1997/1998, 32-35.